Harmony on the Plate

Natural Nutrition for sexual Vitality

Henry L. Duke

Chapter One

Harmony on the Plate for beginners

The book "Harmony on the Plate: Natural Nutrition for Sexual Vitality" explores the complex relationship between nutrition and sexual function. This thorough manual starts out by explaining how nutrition plays a critical part in promoting sexual vitality and stressing the importance of eating a balanced diet to maximize intimate well-being.

The book deftly examines the dietary elements necessary to sustain a strong sexual health regimen. It breaks down the significance of macro- and micronutrients and emphasizes the role that antioxidants, vitamins, and minerals have in promoting sexual vigor. It also emphasizes how important water is for maintaining general physiological processes that are essential for intimacy.

The plethora of foods that are well-known for their aphrodisiac qualities and ability to improve erotic performance are explained to readers. The story emphasizes how important plant-based diets, lean proteins, and healthy fats are for maintaining hormonal balance and maintaining the kind of energy needed for sexual activity.

The book also explores the unique advantages of important nutrients like zinc, vitamin D, and omega-3 fatty acids in enhancing libido and maximizing sexual performance. The significant influence that lifestyle factors such as exercise, stress reduction, and restful sleep have on sexual health is also thoroughly investigated

Beyond just theoretical discussion, "Harmony on the Plate" offers doable meal plans and delicious recipes designed to stimulate sexual libido. In addition, it tackles frequent worries about sexual health, busting myths and providing evidence-based dietary recommendations for reducing common problems.

In the end, "Harmony on the Plate" is a priceless tool for anyone hoping to use the healing potential of whole foods to develop a satisfying and exciting love relationship.

Chapter Two

Significance of Nutrition in sexual health

An individual's libido, reproductive health, and general sexual well-being are all impacted by a number of physiological processes that are influenced by nutrition. The following are some ways that diet affects sexual health:

1. Hormone Regulation: The synthesis and balancing of hormones depend on a number of minerals, including zinc, vitamin D, and omega-3 fatty acids. Key components of sexual desire, arousal, and performance are hormones like progesterone, estrogen, and testosterone.

2. Blood Circulation: Sufficient blood flow to the genitalia is guaranteed by a robust cardiovascular system, which is essential for sexual activity. Foods high in nitric oxide, such as leafy greens and beets, can help widen blood vessels, improving circulation and promoting arousal in women and erections in males.

3. Energy and Stamina: Foods high in nutrients give you the energy you need to engage in sexual activity. Energy levels are maintained by complex carbs, lean proteins, and healthy fats, which promote endurance and stamina during sexual activities.

4. Reproductive Health:

Antioxidants, vitamin E, and folate are among the nutrients that are essential for reproductive health. They boost fertility in men and women, guard against oxidative damage, and aid in the integrity of sperm and eggs.

5. Stress management:

Prolonged stress can impair one's sexual function and desire. Foods high in nutrients, especially those strong in B vitamins and antioxidants, can help reduce oxidative stress and encourage relaxation, which can lessen the negative effects of stress on sexual health.

6. Psychological Well-Being:
Eating habits have an impact on mood, anxiety, and sadness. A strong libido and fulfilling sexual encounters are contingent upon neurotransmitter function and positive mental health, both of which can be enhanced by a well-balanced diet high in omega-3 fatty acids, B vitamins, and magnesium.

7. Body Composition: Sexual health depends on maintaining a healthy body weight and composition. Overweight, particularly in the abdominal area, can throw off the hormone balance and aggravate issues like infertility and erectile dysfunction.

Sexual vitality and health depend on adequate nutrition. A joyful and meaningful sexual life can be fostered by providing the body with a wide variety of nutrient-rich foods, which can also support hormone balance, optimize blood flow, boost energy levels, and promote general well-being.

Chapter Three

Dietary factors that affect sexual arousal

1. Hormonal Balance: The production and balance of hormones are influenced by specific nutrients, which have a direct effect on sexual desire and performance. For instance, women's synthesis of estrogen is influenced by vitamin D, whereas men need zinc to produce testosterone.

2. Blood Circulation: Proper blood flow to the genitalia is encouraged by a diet high in foods that support cardiovascular health, such as fruits, vegetables, healthy grains, and lean meats. This increases arousal and helps women engorge and males achieve erectile function.

3. Energy Levels: Foods high in nutrients provide you the energy you need to engage in sexual activity. Energy levels are maintained by complex carbs, lean proteins, and healthy fats, which promote endurance and stamina during sexual activities.

4. Function of the neurological System: Sexual arousal and pleasure are significantly influenced by the neurological system. B vitamins, magnesium, and omega-3 fatty acids are among the nutrients that enhance

neurotransmitter activity and
proper nerve signaling, which
improves sensitivity and
responsiveness.

5. Reproductive Health:

Fertility and reproductive health
depend on a few key nutrients.
Antioxidants such as vitamin E
and selenium, for instance, shield
eggs and sperm from oxidative
damage, and folate promotes the
formation of healthy embryos and
sperm.

6. Stress management:

Prolonged stress can impair
sexual performance and lower
libido. A diet high in magnesium,
omega-3 fatty acids, and
antioxidants can reduce stress

and encourage relaxation, which improves sexual vigor.

7. Body Composition: Sexual health depends on maintaining a healthy body weight and composition. Overweight can affect sexual function and upset hormone balance, particularly around the abdomen.

8. Psychological Well-Being: Emotion, anxiety, and sadness are all impacted by diet and can have an impact on sexual desire and fulfillment. Eating foods high in nutrients that support brain function, such almonds, leafy greens, and fatty fish, can improve sexual vigor and foster positive mental health.

9. Function of the Endocrine System: The pituitary, thyroid, and adrenal glands are among the glands that make up the endocrine system, which controls the production and reaction of hormones. Tyrosine, selenium, and iodine are among the nutrients that are necessary for optimum endocrine function, which supports sexual health.

10. Function of the Immune System: Sexual and general health are dependent on a robust immune system. Deficits in some nutrients can impair immunity, leaving people more vulnerable to illnesses that might affect fertility and sexual function.

Chapter Four

Understanding Nutrition Requirements for Sexual Vitality:

1. The macronutrients

o **Carbohydrates:** Give you the energy you need for exercise, including sex.

o **Proteins:** Vital for muscle and tissue regeneration, crucial for sexual endurance.

o **Fats:** Essential for the synthesis of hormones and the uptake of fat-soluble vitamins, which impact sexual function and libido.

2. Small-scale nutrients:

o **Vitamins:** Different vitamins are important for neuron function, hormone synthesis, and reproductive health. Vitamin D, B vitamins, and E, for instance, are especially crucial.

o **Minerals:** Selenium promotes sperm motility and antioxidant protection, while zinc is essential for sperm health and testosterone production.

3. Antioxidants

o Guard against oxidative stress, which can harm sexual and reproductive health. Dark leafy greens, almonds, and berries are meals high in antioxidants.

4. Hydration

o **adequate hydration** is

necessary for healthy circulation
and lubrication, two physiological
processes that are critical for
sexual desire and performance.

**Foods to Improve Your Sexual
Health:**

1. Vegetables and Fruits:
o Packed with vitamins, minerals,
and antioxidants that improve
general health and encourage
blood flow.
o Berries, especially those strong
in antioxidants like blueberries
and strawberries, can help with
circulation.
o Nutrients like folate and
magnesium, which support
reproductive health, are found in

leafy greens like spinach and
kale.

2. Whole Grains:

o Provide steady energy and
control blood sugar, both of which
are necessary for preserving
stamina during sex.

o Quinoa, oats, and whole wheat
bread are a few examples.

3. LeanProteins:

o Crucial for hormone synthesis
and muscle regeneration,
promoting sexual performance
and stamina.

o Choose lean sources including
beans, fish, poultry, and tofu.

4. Healthy Fats:

o Omega-3 fatty acids improve
sexual performance by supporting

hormone production and cardiovascular health.

o Include foods like avocados, almonds, seeds, and fatty fish (mackerel, salmon) in your diet.

5. Foods High in Zinc:

o Zinc is essential for healthy sperm and the synthesis of testosterone.

o Include foods high in zinc in your diet, such as red meat, chicken, oysters, nuts, and seeds.

6. Aphrodisiacs:

o There is a long-standing tradition linking specific foods to an increase in libido and sexual desire.

o Dark chocolate, oysters, chile peppers, and watermelon are a few examples.

7. Hydration:

o Maintaining blood volume and lubrication, which promotes sexual desire, requires enough water.

o Include hydrating foods like cucumbers, melons, and citrus fruits in your diet and drink lots of water.

By offering crucial nutrients, stimulating circulation, and improving general wellbeing, including these items in your diet can improve sexual health and vitality.

Chapter Five

The Power of Plant-Based Diets for Sexual Health:

1.Antioxidants

o Antioxidants found in plant-based diets assist in reducing oxidative stress and neutralizing free radicals in all areas of the body, including the reproductive organs.

o Antioxidants shield cells from harm, promoting the general health and functionality of the reproductive system.

2. Production of Nitric Oxide:

o Compounds included in several plant diets encourage the synthesis of nitric oxide, a

chemical that widens blood vessels and enhances blood flow.
o Sexual arousal and performance can be enhanced by increased blood flow to the genitalia.

3. The phytonutrients

o Plants include bioactive substances called phytonutrients, which provide a number of health advantages, including promoting sexual health.

o Some examples are polyphenols, lignans, and flavonoids, which have been linked to enhanced sperm quality, libido, and erectile function.

4. Fiber:

o Dietary fiber, which promotes

digestive health and balances
hormone levels, is abundant in
plant-based diets.

o By increasing satiety and
stabilizing blood sugar levels,
fiber lowers the risk of obesity
and other disorders that may
affect sexual performance.

5. Balance of Hormones:

o Phytoestrogens, or substances
that imitate estrogen in the body,
are present in some plant-based
diets. Despite being debatable,
phytoestrogens may aid in
controlling men's and women's
hormonal balance.

o Retaining libido, fertility, and
general sexual health requires
hormone balance.

6. Heart Conditions:

o Diets based primarily on plants are linked to a decreased risk of hypertension, cardiovascular disease, and other disorders that can affect a person's ability to conceive.

o Plant-based diets indirectly improve sexual vigor by enhancing cardiovascular and blood circulation through the promotion of heart health

Including a range of plant-based foods in your diet, such as whole grains, legumes, nuts, seeds, fruits, and vegetables, can have a positive impact on your general and sexual health.

Chapter Six

Vegetables and fruits that are rich in antioxidants

Antioxidants, which are abundant in fruits and vegetables, are essential for preventing oxidative damage to cells and supporting general health, which includes sexual health. The following are some fruits and vegetables that are high in antioxidants:

1.Berries:

o Blueberries

o Berries

o Berries

o Blackberries

o Cranberries

2.Fruits with Citrus Flavors:

o Oranges

o Grapes

o Lemons

o Limes

3.Tropical Fruits:

o Kiwi

o Papaya

o Pineapple

o Mango

4.Greens with leaves:

o Spinach

o Kale

o Swiss chard

o Collard greens

5.Cruciferous Squash:

o Broccoli

o Cauliflower

o Brussels sprouts

o Cabbage

6.Tomatoes:

o Packed with lycopene, a potent antioxidant linked to better cardiovascular health and possible advantages for the reproductive system in men.

7. Bell Peppers:

o In particular, bell peppers especially red, orange, and yellow ones—are rich in antioxidants and vitamin C.

8.Red and Purple Fruits:

o Pomegranates

o Cherries

o Grapes in red

o Plums

Legumes and whole grains for enduring energy

Excellent providers of complex carbs, fiber, protein, and other micronutrients that promote general health and give prolonged energy are whole grains and legumes. This is how they support long-term energy:

1. Complex carbohydrate:

o Complex carbs are broken down more slowly than simple carbohydrates and are found in whole grains including quinoa, brown rice, oats, and whole wheat.

o Complex carbs give a constant supply of energy by releasing glucose into the bloodstream gradually, avoiding blood sugar spikes and crashes.

2. Fiber:

o Dietary fiber from whole grains and legumes slows down the digestion and absorption of carbs.

o Fiber helps control blood sugar levels, which prevents energy crashes and encourages sustained energy.

3. Protein

o Legumes is a great source of plant-based protein; examples include beans, lentils, and chickpeas.

o Compared to just carbs, protein helps preserve muscle mass and offers a more sustained energy source.

4. Small-scale nutrients:

o Iron, magnesium, zinc, and B vitamins are among the vitamins and minerals that are abundant in whole grains and legumes and are crucial for energy metabolism.

o These micronutrients help the body produce and use energy as efficiently as possible by facilitating the metabolism of proteins, lipids, and carbs into energy.

Chapter Seven

Lean protein consumption for hormone balance and muscle power

Lean protein consumption is crucial for maintaining hormone balance, muscle strength, and general health. The following are the ways that lean proteins support these ideas:

1. Muscle Strength:

o Since proteins are the building blocks of muscle tissue, eating enough of them is essential for keeping and mending muscle fibers.

o Lean proteins offer high-quality protein with little saturated fat. Examples of these are turkey, chicken breast, fish, tofu, and low-fat dairy products.

o Eating lean protein after working out promotes muscle growth and recovery, gradually increasing muscle strength and endurance.

2. Balance of Hormones:

o The synthesis of several hormones, including growth hormone, insulin, and sex hormones like estrogen and testosterone, depends on protein.

o Amino acids, which are found in lean proteins, are building blocks for hormones and neurotransmitters that control mood, energy levels, and sexual activity.

o Eating enough protein promotes hormone balance, which is essential for libido, reproductive health, and general wellbeing.

3. Contentment and Control of Weight:

o Because protein is so satiating, it makes you feel satisfied and full after eating, which lowers the chance of overindulging and helps you maintain a healthy weight.

o Lean proteins can help avoid energy crashes and cravings by boosting feelings of fullness and maintaining blood sugar levels, enabling sustainable energy throughout the day.

4. Density of nutrients:

o Essential vitamins and minerals, including iron, zinc, and B vitamins, which are critical for energy metabolism, immunological response, and hormone synthesis, are also present in lean proteins in addition to being high in protein.
o Including a selection of lean proteins in your diet guarantees that you get all the nutrients required for maximum health and energy.

Good fats and how they affect the synthesis of hormones

Because they supply the building blocks for hormone synthesis and maintain hormone signaling pathways, healthy fats are essential for hormone production and balance. The following are some instances of good fats and how they affect the synthesis of hormones:

1. The Fatty Acids Omega-3:

o Found in walnuts, hemp seeds, flaxseeds, chia seeds, and fatty fish (salmon, mackerel, and sardines).

o The creation of prostaglandins, which control inflammation and hormone synthesis, requires the presence of omega-3 fatty acids.

o They promote cardiovascular

health, mood stability, and healthy brain function—all of which have an impact on hormone balance.

2. Fats Monounsaturated:

o Contains avocados, sesame and pumpkin seeds, olive oil, nuts (such almonds, cashews, and peanuts), and seeds.

o Monounsaturated fats assist in controlling insulin sensitivity, a process critical to blood sugar regulation and hormone homeostasis.

o They support hormone signaling by offering a steady supply of energy and assisting in the preservation of cell membrane integrity.

3. Moderate intake of saturated fats:

o Present in full-fat dairy products, butter from grass-fed cows, and coconut oil.

o Because they act as precursors to steroid hormones like estrogen and testosterone, saturated fats are crucial for the generation of hormones.

o Moderate consumption of saturated fats can promote hormone synthesis and balance; however, excessive consumption may have detrimental effects on health.

A diverse range of healthful fats can be included in your diet to assist hormone production and balance, which will benefit your general health and wellbeing. To make sure you get a balanced amount of important fatty acids required for healthy hormone activity, try to incorporate sources of omega-3 fatty acids, monounsaturated fats, and saturated fats in your meals.

Chapter Eight

Particular Nutrients and Their Advantages

Without a doubt, the following nutrients are crucial for sexual health and have advantages:

1. Zinc

o Advantages: Men's synthesis of testosterone, which promotes sperm health and libido, depends on it. Zinc helps women regulate their ovulation and menstrual periods.

o Food Sources: Whole grains, legumes, nuts, seeds, chicken, red meat, and oysters.

2. The Fatty Acids Omega-3:

o Advantages: Promote

cardiovascular health, enhance vaginal blood flow, and control hormone production. They also lessen inflammation and improve mood.

o Food Sources: walnuts, hemp seeds, flaxseeds, chia seeds, and fatty fish (salmon, mackerel, and sardines).

3. Vitamin D

o Advantages: Aids in the synthesis of testosterone, boosts immunity, and preserves bone health. The regularity of menstruation and estrogen levels in women might be impacted by vitamin D levels.

o Food Sources: Sunlight exposure, egg yolks, fortified

plant-based milk, dairy products, and fatty fish.

4. Vitamin E

o Advantages: Serves as an antioxidant to shield cells from oxidative harm. Through its ability to shield sperm and egg cells from free radicals, it promotes reproductive health.

o Food sources include avocado, spinach, nuts (almonds, hazelnuts, and sunflower seeds), and seeds (pumpkin seeds, among others).

5. Vitamin B:

o Advantages: Vital for hormone synthesis, neuronal function, and energy metabolism. B vitamins are important for mood modulation and neurotransmitter synthesis. In particular, B6, B9 (folate), and B12 are important.

o Food Sources: Fish, poultry, eggs, dairy products, legumes, nuts, seeds, and leafy greens.

6. The mineral magnesium

o Advantages: Promotes blood sugar regulation, helps with energy metabolism, and supports muscle and nerve function. Additionally, magnesium may lessen stress and enhance sleep, which may have a knock-on effect on sexual health.

o Food Sources: legumes, whole grains, almonds, peanuts, cashews, and spinach.

Factors related to lifestyle

Undoubtedly, a person's lifestyle has a big impact on their sexual health and vigor. The following are some crucial aspects of lifestyle to think about:

1. Exercise:

o Frequent exercise increases vitality, enhances blood circulation, and supports cardiovascular health all of which are critical for sexual performance.

o Moreover, exercise improves mood, lowers stress levels, and boosts confidence—elements that have a favorable effect on libido and sexual satisfaction.

2. Handling Stress:

o Prolonged stress has a deleterious effect on arousal, performance, and sexual desire. Developing appropriate coping mechanisms for stress, such as hobbies, mindfulness exercises, and relaxation techniques, can enhance general wellbeing and sexual health.

o Getting assistance from friends, relatives, or a therapist as well as talking to a spouse can also help reduce stress and improve close connections.

3. Restful Sleep:

o For general health and wellbeing, including sexual health, enough sleep is crucial.

Weak sleep or insufficient sleep can cause a reduction in libido, irritability, and exhaustion.

o Better sleep and increased sexual vigor can be achieved by establishing a regular sleep pattern, developing a calming nighttime ritual, and furnishing a comfortable sleeping environment.

4. Wholesome connections

o A fulfilling and happy sexual relationship is facilitated by open communication and strong emotional ties.

o Developing closeness, trust, and respect for one another creates a safe space for enjoying and exploring sexuality.

5. Use of Substances:

o Overindulgence in drugs, smoking, and drinking can eventually lower libido and affect sexual function.

o Reducing or abstaining from these substances can assist preserve sexual health and shield against long-term issues.

6. Body Image and Self-Care:

o Developing a favorable body image and engaging in self-care can boost one's sexual happiness and self-confidence.

o Exercise, hobbies, and self-expression are examples of activities that boost self-esteem and can support a positive sense of self as well as enhanced sexual health.

7. Exploration and Education on Sexuality:

o Gaining knowledge about sexual health, consent, and pleasure can enable people to explore their desires in a respectful and safe way and make educated decisions.

o Intimacy and increased sexual satisfaction are fostered by open conversation about sexual preferences, boundaries, and concerns with partners.

People can enhance their general well-being, sexual health, and vitality by giving this lifestyle aspects top priority and making wise decisions.

Chapter Nine

Recipes and Meal Plans

Recipes and Meal Plans for Sexual Wellness:

Day1:

• Greek yogurt parfait with almonds and mixed berries for breakfast

• Quinoa salad for lunch, topped with avocado, cherry tomatoes, grilled chicken, spinach, and lemon vinaigrette

• Snack: Almond butter on sliced apples

• Supper is baked salmon paired with sweet potato wedges and roasted asparagus.

Day 2:

- Omelettes with spinach and mushrooms and whole grain toast for breakfast.
- For lunch, try this: lentil soup paired with a mixed green salad dressed with a balsamic vinaigrette, cucumbers, and chickpeas.
- Snack: Hummus-topped carrot sticks
- Dinner is brown rice, broccoli, bell peppers, and snap peas stir-fried with grilled tofu.

Day 3:

- Oatmeal prepared the night before with rolled oats, almond milk, chia seeds, banana slices, and honey drizzled on top.
- Lunch consists of a whole wheat

wrap with spinach, hummus, and grilled veggies.

• Snack: Greek yogurt topped with a cinnamon sprinkle and a mixture of nuts.

• Dinner is turkey meatballs with steamed broccoli on the side and whole wheat spaghetti with marinara sauce.

Day 4:

• Smoothie for breakfast consisting of banana, pineapple, kale, spinach, Greek yogurt, and coconut water

• Quinoa and black bean salad paired with red onion, cilantro, maize, cherry tomatoes, and lime-cumin dressing for lunch.

• Snack: Pear slices with honey

drizzled over and ricotta cheese

• Dinner is quinoa pilaf and grilled chicken breast with roasted Brussels sprouts.

Day 5:

• Avocado toast with cherry tomatoes and poached eggs for breakfast

• For lunch, try a chickpea salad topped with cucumber, olives, feta cheese, mixed greens, and a lemon-tahini dressing.

• Snack: Peach slices with cottage cheese and a dash of cinnamon

• Supper is baked cod paired with roasted carrots and a quinoa tabbouleh salad.

Dietary Guidelines for Frequently Seen Sexual Health Problems:

1. ED, or erectile dysfunction:

o Eat antioxidant-rich foods to support vascular health and blood flow, such as leafy greens, citrus fruits, and berries.

o Include foods rich in omega-3 fatty acids, such as walnuts, flaxseeds, and fatty fish, to promote heart health and lower inflammation.

o Reduce your intake of processed foods, sugar-filled drinks, and high-fat foods as these can aggravate diabetes, obesity, and heart problems linked to ED.

o Eat more nitrate-rich foods, such as leafy greens and beets, as these can enhance erectile function and blood vessel dilatation.

2. Low libido

o To enhance testosterone production and libido, eat foods high in zinc, such as oysters, red meat, poultry, nuts, and seeds.

o Include meals strong in vitamin D, such as fatty fish, dairy products with added fortification, and time spent in the sun, since low libido has been related to vitamin D insufficiency.

o Include meals high in B vitamins, such as legumes, whole grains, and leafy greens, to enhance mood and energy levels, as these can affect libido

Steer clear of excessive alcohol intake since it might lower libido and affect sexual performance.

3. Ejaculation prematurely (PE):

o Eat foods high in magnesium to enhance nervous system function and lower stress, which may be a contributing factor to PE. Examples of such foods include leafy greens, nuts, seeds, and whole grains.

o Add meals high in serotonin precursors, including almonds, turkey, and bananas, to help regulate your mood and maybe postpone ejaculation o Restrict your caffeine intake because too much of it can make you more anxious and lead to PE.

o Use relaxing methods to reduce stress and anxiety related to PE, such as deep breathing exercises and meditation.

4. Irregularities in menstruation:

o Eat meals high in iron, such as leafy greens, lean meats, legumes, and fortified cereals, to maintain iron levels and lower the chance of irregular menstruation brought on by iron deficiency.

o Include foods strong in vitamin C, like bell peppers, citrus fruits, and strawberries, to improve the absorption of iron from plant-based sources.

Incorporate foods high in omega-3 fatty acids, such as chia seeds, flaxseeds, and fatty fish, to maintain hormonal balance and reduce inflammation.

o Reduce your intake of processed foods, sugary snacks, and coffee because these items might make menstruation abnormalities and hormone imbalances worse.

When treating common sexual health concerns, these dietary considerations can be used in conjunction with other therapy modalities and lifestyle changes. For tailored food guidance and treatment suggestions, it's crucial

to speak with a medical
practitioner or certified dietician.

9 798328 109192